# YOUR KNOWLEDGE HAS VALUE

- We will publish your bachelor's and master's thesis, essays and papers

- Your own eBook and book - sold worldwide in all relevant shops

- Earn money with each sale

Upload your text at www.GRIN.com and publish for free

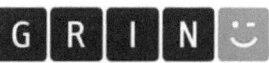

Geffrey Li

# Cost-effectiveness analysis of HIV/AIDS "Test and treat" strategy vs. Current treatment guideline in Botswana

GRIN Publishing

**Bibliographic information published by the German National Library:**

The German National Library lists this publication in the National Bibliography; detailed bibliographic data are available on the Internet at http://dnb.dnb.de .

**Imprint:**

Copyright © 2015 GRIN Verlag GmbH
Print and binding: Books on Demand GmbH, Norderstedt Germany
ISBN: 978-3-656-92165-3

**This book at GRIN:**

http://www.grin.com/en/e-book/294007/cost-effectiveness-analysis-of-hiv-aids-test-and-treat-strategy-vs

**GRIN - Your knowledge has value**

Since its foundation in 1998, GRIN has specialized in publishing academic texts by students, college teachers and other academics as e-book and printed book. The website www.grin.com is an ideal platform for presenting term papers, final papers, scientific essays, dissertations and specialist books.

**Visit us on the internet:**

http://www.grin.com/

http://www.facebook.com/grincom

http://www.twitter.com/grin_com

# Cost-effectiveness analysis of HIV/AIDS "Test and treat" strategy vs. Current treatment guideline in Botswana

Geffrey Nan Li, MD, MSPH

Johns Hopkins Bloomberg School of Public Health

**Summary**

A more aggressive strategy "test and treat" is predicted to reduce AIDS-related mortality, increase the life expectancy of people living with HIV and is cost-effective. However, the cost-effectiveness studies related to "test and treat" strategy did not consider the possibility of increased drug resistance due to poor adherence, which is not rare in developing countries. There is a need for a cost-effectiveness analysis related to "test and treat" strategy in developing countries that includes drug resistance as an important parameter. This analysis is to support the government of Botswana to examine the cost-effectiveness of a HIV/AIDS "test and treat" strategy vs. current treatment guideline, which is providing treatment to patients with a CD4 count of <350 cells/ µL.

**Objective:** Compare "test and treat" strategy regardless of CD4 level and the current guideline of initiation with CD4 ≤350 cells/µL for HIV-infected adults in Botswana, taking drug resistance as an important parameter.

**Methods:** This analysis was done using Markov model with a cohort of 10,000 healthy people from a governmental perspective. Data was obtained from published clinical, epidemiological, and economic journals as well as reports released by Botswana government and other international organizations. When possible, parameters were estimated based on Botswana settings.

**Results:** The total costs were $ 2934261.67 for "test and treat" strategy and $ 2676606.19 for the current treatment guideline in ten years. The QALYs for "test and treat" strategy and for the current treatment guideline are 20923.17 years and 20515.43 years. Compared with current treatment guideline, "test and treat" gained 407.74 QALYs. The incremental cost-effectiveness ratio (ICER) of "test and treat" versus current treatment guideline was $ 631.91 per QALY.

Based on one-way sensitivity analysis, changing the value of incidence under "test and treat" strategy and treatment coverage among HIV infected population under both strategies will significantly influence ICER. Variations in the MDR rate, cost of first line and second line treatment, annual discount rate will have moderate impacts on ICER.

**Conclusions**: "Test and treat" strategy for adult individuals (>16 years old) regardless CD4 level is very cost-effective. Drug resistance and ART cost have moderate impact on ICER. Incidence and treatment coverage among HIV infected population are the main drivers of ICER. For Botswana, "test and treat" strategy for adult population should be considered.

# Contents

**Chapter 1: Introduction: Research background and rationale**

Acquired immunodeficiency syndrome (AIDS) has killed more than 25 million people since 1981, and about 33 million people (most of them living in low- and middle-income countries) are now infected with human immunodeficiency virus (HIV) [1].

As one of the major treatments against HIV/AIDS, highly active antiretroviral therapy (ART) became available in 1996 but was extremely expensive in developing countries. Lack of ART in developing countries was a problem and was declared as a global health emergency in 2003, since then governments, international agencies, and funding bodies began to implement plans to increase ART coverage in low and mid-income countries. In 2009, more than a third of people who needed ART were receiving it [2].

HIV destroys immune system cells such as CD4 T-cells, leaving infected individuals susceptible to other infections. The CD4 T-cell count (CD4 count) is the major laboratory indicator of immune function in patients who have HIV infection, and it is one of the key factors in determining urgency of ART initiation. For most low and mid-income countries, CD4 count measurements play an important role in determining eligibility for ART [3]. In 2013, World Health Organization released a more aggressive guideline compared to previous guidelines on the use of antiretroviral drugs for treating and preventing HIV infection, which encouraged early treatment for patients with a CD4 cell amount less than 500 cells per cubic millimeter (cells/μL). [3] This is also known as "early treatment", which defined as therapy initiated when the CD4+ T-cell count ranged from 350 to 500 cells/μL.

The reason why WHO released a more aggressive ART guideline was because the median baseline CD4 count at which people initiate ART has been suggested to be risen during the past decade by a lot of research evidence [4-10]. In 2003 Velasco-Hernandez and colleagues were the first to propose that treatment could potentially be used to eliminate HIV epidemics. Different from early treatment, "test and treat" is a more aggressive strategy and predicted by the modeling that if everyone is tested regularly and all infected persons are put on ART regardless of CD4 level, HIV/AIDS can be eliminated from society [4].

The reasons for the decline of HIV/AIDS prevalence in some "test and treat" modeling [5-10] are: (1) Clinical trial findings demonstrates that probability of HIV transmission was reduced under "test and treat" strategy [5-8], since initiation of ART at early stages of the disease can reduce the plasma viral load by up to six orders of magnitude [4]. (2) Evidence suggests that testing HIV positive causes dramatic reductions in sexual activity levels, which also reduces HIV transmission probability [9, 10]. But others also find that benefits from expanded ART use are counterbalanced by modest increases in risky sexual behavior [11-13].

As for the degree of the decline of HIV/AIDS prevalence, existing mathematical models that simulate the impact of scaling up "test-and-treat" policies show mixed results. Some find significant gains in averting new HIV infections for more aggressive treatment strategies [14-16], whereas others find only modest effects [17-18].

4

Instability of the models and the discrepancy in model findings in "test and-treat" outcomes reflect the sensitivity of assumptions about HIV prevalence and other population parameters. This highlights the need to calibrate mathematical models to mimic the real world HIV prevalence trends [19].

Actually, the potential benefits of "test and treat" strategy are not limited to the reduction of AIDS epidemic. Recent economic analysis found that investment in antiretroviral therapy is cost-effective and may also result in cost savings [20-21]. The cost savings of HIV/AIDS treatment is very important to the world, since the spending in HIV/AIDS prevention and treatment is tremendous. In 2011, an estimated US$16.8 billion was spent on HIV/AIDS, compared to US$ 300 million in 1996. This is also an 11 percent increase on the money spent on HIV and AIDS in 2010 [2]. The spending is still estimated to be increasing. In Hecht R's modeling, without a serious change in approach, AIDS will still be a major pandemic and the funding required in resource-poor countries could reach an estimated $35 billion annually by 2031, which is two times more than the current level [22]. It is important to include costing into the model when conducting analysis for different HIV treatment and prevent strategies. Also, for public health officials and policy makers in general to make a determination about the validity and feasibility of a "test and treat" strategy, biomedical findings must be linked to costing.

The reason why "test and treat" could be cost-saving is that investment in HIV treatment could increase employment and productivity and also avert future expenses for medical expenditure. [23]. Cost-effectiveness studies have been done around cost-effectiveness of "test and treat" strategies. Some are focusing on impact of "test" [24][25], and some are only focusing on expanding treatment to larger population [26]. One cost-effectiveness of HIV testing and treatment model in South Africa showed that increasing the length of the survival time, although beneficial to individuals, reduces the probability of eliminating HIV and decreases the cost-effectiveness of using universal "test and treat" strategies [27].

The studies of cost-effectiveness analysis for "test and treat" strategies are limited. There are some cost-effectiveness analysis for early ART. One early ART in persons infected with HIV in serodiscordant couples was conducted in South Africa and India settings, using a computer simulation of the progression of HIV infection. The results show that early ART is very cost-effective over a lifetime under most modeled assumptions in the two countries [20]. Another cost-effectiveness of early ART used multiple independent mathematical models to evaluate the potential health impact, costs, and cost-effectiveness on different adult ART eligibility criteria. The study is from a health system perspective with results projected over 20 years in four settings—South Africa, Zambia, India, and Vietnam. And results show earlier ART eligibility can be very cost-effective in low and middle-income settings [21].

However, drug resistance is an issue that could potentially counterbalance the cost savings. Velasco-Hernandez and colleagues also noted that the emergence of highly transmissible resistant strains of HIV can significantly reduce the benefits of early ART [28]. Baggaley et al also found that early treatment is ineffective as a measure to control sub-Saharan African HIV epidemics, as increasing the proportion on treatment increases the emergence and spread of multiple-drug-resistant HIV (MDR) [29].

Potential effects of MDR under "test and treat" strategy can be further divided into two parts. The first part is the effect of higher coverage of ART. Expanding eligibility for use of ART will result in higher coverage of ART in HIV-infected population, which could cause more patients generate MDR due to poor adherence especially in developing countries. This treatment failure will bring more cost burden, since more patients will move from first-line treatment to second-line treatment, and in some African countries, the price of second line drugs could be much more expensive than the first line drugs [30]. The second part is the effect of higher prevalence of MDR. Sood et al's mathematical modeling indicated that "test and treat" could lead to even a near doubling of the prevalence of MDR (9.06% compared to 4.79%) in 10 years under 'test and treat' policy [31]. Higher rates of MDR will counterbalance the benefit of HIV infections averted by "test and treat" strategy.

However, Gonzalez-Serna criticized Sood et al's result, "even if the estimates of Sood et al for MDR in their model were correct and the proportion of cases of MDR would increase, the total number of cases of MDR would increase only slightly." [32] The effects of MDR on cost-effectiveness of "test and treat" strategy remains controversial. In addition, most cost-effectiveness studies did not explicitly address potential effects of MDR under "test and treat" strategy, which is not rare in developing countries due to poor adherence [33]. There is a need for a cost-effectiveness study related to "test and treat" in developing countries that includes drug resistance as an important parameter.

## Botswana

### Profile of the Republic of Botswana
Botswana is a land-locked country in southern Africa with a population of 1.7 million people. The rate of economic growth in Botswana has been increasing in recent years, due to democratic governance and rich mineral resources, making Botswana a middle-income country. Total GDP of Botswana grew at an annual rate of 8% from 1999 to 2005[34]. Botswana has experienced significant progress both in economics and equity. The government has also placed much attention on health issues; many organizations are involved in promoting population health.

### The HIV epidemic in Botswana
The major disease burden in Botswana is from infectious diseases with the HIV prevalence rate in the general population of Botswana at 17.1%. This is among the highest HIV prevalence in the world [35]. HIV/AIDS has a large impact on adult mortality rate in Botswana: (1) Between 1980 and 1997, both male and female life expectancy declined in Botswana (61% and 51% respectively), mainly because of high HIV prevalence [36]. There is also a heavy impact on population health, especially for young women and pregnant women, age 20-34. (2) HIV/AIDS influences the social and economic fronts of life in Botswana, and this is due to the disease burden and its impact in terms of costs managing of the disease as well as the impact on the overall well-being of the people. [34]

### Response to the HIV epidemic
Botswana has made significant progress toward the reduction of HIV transmission in its population through many programs, mass mobilization and education efforts. The government

and other organizations have carried out many programs to treat HIV/AIDS patients and implemented HIV/AIDS prevention intervention programs.

For examples, Botswana has provided HIV testing to the general population free of charge and routinely at all clinics. Also Botswana was the first country in Africa to launched a program, known as the MASA ART program ("Masa" is a Setswana word meaning "a new dawn"), to try to provide access to HIV drug treatment nationwide since 2002. Free ART and rapid expansion of HIV services over the past decades enabled the number of people receiving ART to increase several fold by the end of 2012. Today, more than 95 percent of all adults and children eligible for treatment are receiving it [37].

However, Botswana is still facing the challenge of having one of the highest prevalence of HIV/AIDS in the world and its HIV prevalence rates have stabilized in recent years. Finding other more effective and preventative measures is essential. Facing these challenges, whether Botswana should move toward a more progressive ART strategy as suggested by WHO HIV treatment guideline remains a question. (Current national treatment guideline of Botswana recommends providing treatment to patients with a CD4 count of <350 cells/ μL.)

**Cost-effectiveness analysis in Markov model**
We established a cost-effectiveness analysis for different ART strategies, which is based on a Markov model. Our study will include HIV/AIDS drug resistance as an important parameter, which could lead to a failure of a proportion of treatment, making patients move from first-line treatment to the second-line treatment. As a result, patients are split into different treatment phases, therefore multi-state models should be adopted in this analysis. Multi-state models could help with estimation of proportions of individuals who will be in the various states at some time in the future, providing a comprehensive view of a disease process [38].
Multi-state Markov models can be very useful in this cost-effectiveness analysis: (1) States will be explicitly accounted and based on treatment phases; (2) Also patients could live with HIV for a long time if they are on treatments, so costs and effects spread over a long period of time should be measured by Markov model.

Our study contributes to literature by using a Markov model to simulate effects of "test and treat" for the adult AIDS patients. First, most cost-effectiveness studies did not explicitly address potential effects of the spread of MDR due to poor adherence under "test and treat" policies in a mid-income country. Second, no previous study has focused on "test-and-treat" in Botswana, a mid-income country with a high prevalence of 17.1% [35] and where patients have universal access to the free ART. The results could help inform policy makers on where to focus future HIV prevention efforts.

7

**Chapter 2: Study objectives**

1. To support Botswana government examining the cost-effectiveness of a HIV/AIDS "test and treat" strategy VS current treatment guideline.
2. Assess the impact of drug resistance on the HIV/AIDS "test and treat" strategy.


**Chapter 3: Study design and methodology**
**a. Study design**
Our study examined the cost-effectiveness of a HIV/AIDS "test and treat" strategy versus current treatment guideline in Botswana from a governmental perspective, since our audience is Botswana government. Cost-effectiveness analysis was based on a Markov model (figure 1).

**Figure 1 Markov Model**

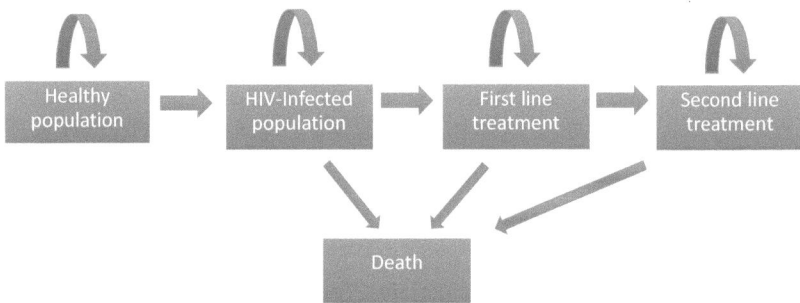

We used a Microsoft Excel based Markov model to evaluate the impact and cost-effectiveness of "test and treat" strategy in Botswana by comparing HIV/AIDS disease and cost burden for two strategies: (1) "Test and treat" strategy regardless of CD4 level; (2) Botswana current guideline, which is initiation of ART for adults with CD4 ≤350 cells/µL.

Health states include healthy population, HIV-infected population without treatment, HIV-infected patients on the first line treatment, HIV-infected patients on the second line treatment, and death. Individuals start initially in a "healthy" state, in time, some may enter a "HIV-infected" state, after that some will get on the "first-line treatment" state. When drug resistance happens, some patients will move to the "second-line treatment" state. "Death" state is an absorbing state.

As one of the processes before ART treatment as well as major expenses included in "test and treat" strategy, HIV testing coverage however does not have a major impact on the comparison between "test and treat" and current treatment strategies under Botswana settings, since the percentage of adults who received a HIV test in 2013 and were informed of the results is from 96.7-97.5% [39] in Botswana. So we didn't include HIV test as a state in this model. The high coverage of HIV test might be the achievements of Botswana government providing HIV test to the general population routinely and free of charge at all clinics.

This analysis was done on a cohort of 10,000 healthy people. Our analytical horizon for examine the disease burden is a 10-year period because we will use the MDR rate from Sood et al's mathematical modeling 9.1% in 10 years after "test and treat" policy. Our study was simulated with 1-year base transition cycle.

We measured the cost-effectiveness in 2013 US dollars per quality-adjusted life-year (QALYs). Main model inputs included measures of disease burden (measured by QALYs for HIV-infected population, AIDS patients on the first-line treatment and AIDS patients on the second-line treatment), possibilities of transitions of different AIDS stages, HIV/AIDS prevalence, direct treatment costs (cost of first-line treatment and second-line treatment), and related cost.

### b. Data Source
Table one (see below) shows the epidemiological parameters and economic parameters we used to estimate the principle base-case values, sensitivity ranges, and references and assumptions of model inputs for estimating impact and cost-effectiveness of the program, respectively. The data in Table 1 is based on the population or average value of the population, not individual level.

**Table 1 Key model parameters with source and ranges**
**(Clinical Events and Transition Probabilities, Annual costs to government)**

| Parameter | Value | Range | Source |
|---|---|---|---|
| **Clinical Events and Transition Probabilities (%) year bases** | | | |
| Incidence of AIDS in adults (CD 350) | 2.92 | N.A. | [39] |
| Incidence of AIDS in adults (Treat all) | 2.19 EST | (1.75, 2.74) | [15] [40] [41][42] |
| Initial access to first-line treatment (CD 350) | 48 EST | (36,60) | [43] [44] [45] |
| Probability of adult AIDS patients moving from first-line to the second line (350) | 4.79 EST | (3.59, 5.60) | [19] [46] [47] |
| Probability of adult AIDS patients moving from first-line to the second line (Treat all) | 7.00 EST | (5.25,8.75) | [19] |
| Probability of death for adult AIDS patients when they are on first-line treatment (CD 350) | 0.30 | (0.23, 0.38) | [48] |
| Probability of death for adult AIDS patients when they are on second-line treatment each year (CD 350) | 0.15 | (0.11,0.19) | [48] |
| Probability of death for adult AIDS patients when they are on first-line treatment (Treat all) | 0.18 | (0.14, 0.23) | [49] |
| Probability of death for adult AIDS patients when they are on second-line treatment each year (Treat all) | 0.09 | (0.068, 0.11) | [49] |
| Probability of death for HIV-infected population who are not on treatment | 9.3 EST | (7.0, 11.6) | [50] |
| **Annual costs per patient to government (US$)** | | | |

9

| Cost of laboratory tests, human resources, opportunistic infections diagnosis and treatment, and infrastructure | 243 | N.A. | [51] |
|---|---|---|---|
| First-line regimen-drugs only | 153 | N.A. | [52] |
| Second-line drug regimen-drugs only | 463 | N.A. | [52] |
| **QALYs** | | | |
| Preference weight - healthy population | 1 | | |
| Preference weight - HIV-infected patients without treatment | 0.72 | N.A. | [53] |
| Preference weight - HIV-infected patients on the first line treatment | 0.84 | N.A. | [54] |
| Preference weight - HIV-infected patients on the second line treatment | 0.84 | N.A. | [54] |

**Clinical events and transition probabilities**

Epidemiologic and clinical variables considered in the analysis are listed in Table 1. For current guideline scenario, incidence of AIDS in adults, coverage of first-line treatment, probability of adult AIDS patients moving from first-line to the second line, and mortality before and after initiation of treatment are all from recently published or released documents in Botswana, including government report, such as the fourth Botswana HIV/AIDS Impact Survey IV (BAIS VI) as well as other published literatures. For "test and treat" scenario, we used several results from previous mathematical modeling analysis to make estimations.

Probability of death for HIV-infected population who are not on treatment is estimated based on an effectiveness study of HIV cohort study in India, since no related data is available for Botswana. MDR rate is estimated based on Sood N et al's mathematical model of "test and treat" for the population of men who have sex with men in Los Angeles County. Since HIV prevalence, HIV testing rate [35] and ART coverage are similar for Botswana and MSM in LA, also there's no other data source for MDR rate under "test and treat" policy.

**Annual costs to government (US$)**

Principal cost drivers in MASA are from the following major categories: ART drugs, laboratory tests, human resources, opportunistic infections diagnosis and treatment, and infrastructure. The total annual per AIDS patient cost to Botswana Government excluding drugs is $243 [47]. Unit cost of first-line and second-line drug is $ 153 and $ 463 [48].

**QALYs**

Incremental cost can readily be measured in dollars, but to compare different strategies leading diverse health consequences, the health outcomes must be measured in broadly applicable units. In cost-effectiveness analysis, health outcomes are not commonly measuring the increases in survival but improvements in clinical health, which are weighted according to a preference-based measure of well-being [55]. We used QALY to measure the health outcomes. The values are from published literature [53, 54], with 3% annual discounting of future costs and effects, in accordance with WHO criteria.

**Discounting**
Discounting future costs means the opportunity to invest present money, with a 3% annual discount rate applied.

Costing per QALY averted ($/QALY) is the basis of comparison. Following standard benchmarks proposed in international work on cost-effectiveness, we compared the ICER to thresholds for cost-effectiveness defined in reference to the annual gross domestic product (GDP) per capita in each country. Interventions are considered to be highly cost-effective when they have ICERs that fall below the annual per-capita GDP, and are regarded as being potentially cost-effective if they have ICERs between one and three times annual per-capita GDP [56].

**Chapter 4: Results**

**Table 2. Estimated Costs (USD) of "test and treat" related cost**
**Versus current guideline\***

|  | Current guideline | Test and treat | Difference |
|---|---|---|---|
| First-line related cost | 2215478.84 | 2208929.91 | 6548.93 |
| Second-line related cost | 461127.35 | 725331.76 | -264204.41 |
| Total cost | 2676606.19 | 2934261.67 | -257655.48 |

Treatment related costs are discounted with a 3% discount rate.
Setting the annual discounting rate to 0.03, under "test and treat" strategy, first-line treatment related cost will save $ 6548.93, and second-line will cost $ 264204.41 more compared to the current guideline. The total costs were $ 2934261.67 for "test and treat" strategy and $ 2676606.19 for the current treatment guideline in ten years. Overall, "Test and treat" will cost $ 257655.48 more than current guideline. (Table 2)

**Table 3. Estimated Health Outcomes of "test and treat"**
**Versus current guideline**

|  | Current guideline | Test and treat | Difference |
|---|---|---|---|
| Healthy | 18590.47 | 21773.27 | -3182.8 |
| Infected | 612.92 | 302.61 | 310.31 |
| First-line | 1174.88 | 1171.40 | 3.48 |
| Second-line | 137.16 | 215.75 | -78.59 |
| Dead | 0 | 0 | 0 |
| Total | 20515.43 | 20923.17 | -407.74 |

Table 3 shows the QALYs for "test and treat" strategy and for the current treatment guideline were 20923.17 years and 20515.43 years, and compared with current treatment guideline, "test and treat" gained 407.74 QALYs. Of note, the major saving is from healthy population which is 3182.8 QALYs.

**Table 4. Incremental Cost-Effectiveness Ratio (ICER) of "test and treat"**
**Versus current guideline**

|  | Total cost | Incremental cost | Total effect | Incremental effect | ICER |
|---|---|---|---|---|---|
| Current guideline | 2676606.19 |  | 20515.43 |  |  |
| Test and treat | 2934261.67 | 20515.43 | 20923.17 | 407.74 | 631.91 |

Table 4 shows the cost-effectiveness results. The incremental cost-effectiveness ratio (ICER) of "test and treat" versus current treatment guideline was $ 631.91 per QALY. According to WHO thresholds, based on the GDP per capita of $ 16104.91 in Botswana [57], "test and treat" strategy for adult individuals (>16 years old) regardless CD4 level was very cost-effective.

**Chapter 5: Sensitivity Analysis**
To assess the overall robustness of our model and to identify influential parameters for which better empirical data is needed, we performed a one-way sensitivity analysis by varying a single input parameter throughout its range of possible values while keeping all other parameters at their base case. The sensitivity analysis determined which variables have the largest influence on the ICER.

Variables included the costs in two scenarios: first-line and second line cost (low = 50% of base case cost, high = 200% of base case cost); Confidence intervals for other probabilities were used when provided by the source articles. Otherwise, we varies 25% change.

A tornado diagram (figure 2) was used to display the range of ICERs as a result of several one-way sensitivity analyses, with the most influential parameter at the top and moving down in order of importance. All variables that have significant impacts on costs and/or other probabilities were included in the sensitivity analyses. Only the most influential variables were shown in the diagram.

**Figure 2: Tornado diagram**

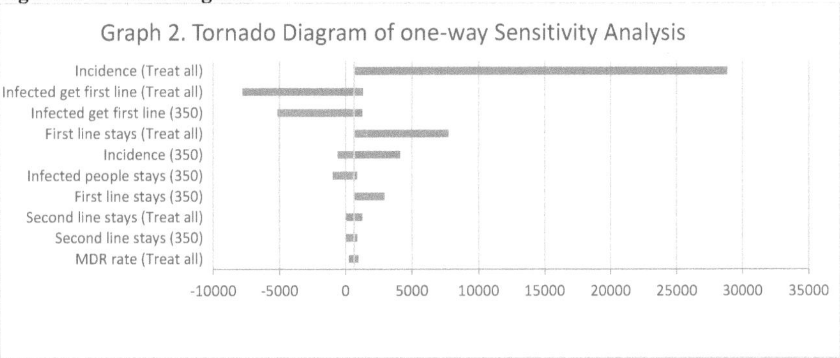

Graph 2. Tornado Diagram of one-way Sensitivity Analysis

Based on sensitivity analysis, changing the value of incidence under "test and treat" strategy and treatment coverage among HIV infected population under both strategies will significantly influence ICER. Variations in the MDR rate, cost of first line and second line treatment, annual discount rate will have moderate impacts on ICER.

## Chapter 6: Conclusions and discussion

In this study, we investigated the potential cost effectiveness of "test and treat" strategy, which is to scale up ART, regardless of AIDS patients' CD 4 count to decrease HIV load at the population level. Based on the GDP per capita of $ 16104.91 in Botswana, our model predicted that the "test and treat" strategy for adult individuals (>16 years old) regardless CD4 count level is very cost-effective (according to WHO thresholds). Drug resistance, ART cost only had a moderate impacts on ICER, while incidence and treatment coverage among HIV infected population had higher impact on ICER. For Botswana, "test and treat" strategy for adult population should be considered.

Our model produced consistent evidence regarding the cost-effectiveness of early ART on the spread of HIV [20-21, 26]. Also, previous studies have raised concerns regarding the impact of drug resistance on cost-effectiveness of early treatment [28] [29]. Our model showed that MDR had only a moderate impact and it was not the main driver of ICER. This proved Gonzalez-Serna's idea that even though the proportion of cases of MDR would increase, the total number of cases of MDR will only increase slightly [33]. This was because "test and treat" strategy reduced the incidence, therefore total number of new infections was decreased in 10 years. We believe our study is the first cost-effectiveness analysis under "test and treat" strategy in a developing country which included drug resistance as an important parameter.

However, limitations of our analysis are important to note. First, some data including MDR rates under "test and treat" strategy is not empirical and is based on mathematical modeling or several estimations, since it is not available in literature. (1) MDR rate. The data we used based on the Sood N and colleagues' modeling could overestimate the impact of MDR on the cost-effectiveness analysis. However in our study, this may not be very significant, because MDR only had only a moderate impact to the cost-effectiveness. (2) Incidence. Although most studies support that increased use of ART could lead to a decrease in HIV incidence, the magnitude of the effect remains poorly characterized, so we estimated it based on several recently published literatures. These unreliable data will decrease the accuracy of the results produced by our model. From the sensitivity analysis we performed on parameters affecting the cost-effectiveness different strategies, we found that the value of incidence will significantly influence ICER. More substantial studies would be needed to provide accurate data to determine impact of "test and treat" strategy on HIV/AIDS incidence.

In order to consider the impact of "test and treat" strategy on transmission, we lowered the incidence in our model. However, we still failed to simulate the transmission mechanism including increased behavioral disinhibition [5-8, 11-13].

Our model showed that "test and treat" is very cost-effective for the government. Also, from a policy perspective, this could also benefit individuals by prolonging their lives. However, the successful implementation of these programs relies on the capacity of overcoming many obstacles to increase access to ART, especially in the rural area of Botswana. The assumptions about scaling up ART access will require a substantial budget investment, intensified community participation, human resources and delivery system. Our analysis cannot determine whether these resources would be available, only that "test and treat" investments provide greater returns than current guideline.

## Acknowledgement

I would like to thank Dr. Heston Philips, Dr. Abdulgafoor Bachani and Dr. David Bishai for their expert advice and encouragement throughout this analysis, as well as my friend Miss Mo Zhou and Miss Guiru Dingfor their both valuable technical and logistical support. I am grateful to UNAIDS and Johns Hopkins University Bloomberg School of Public Health for all of the help they have provided to me.

# Reference

[1] UNAIDS. Global report: UNAIDS report on the global AIDS epidemic 2013, 2013. http://www.unaids.org/en/media/unaids/contentassets/documents/epidemiology/2013/gr2013/UN AIDS_Global_Report_2013_en.pdf. Accessed by April 20th, 2014.

[2] http://www.avert.org/funding-hiv-and-aids.htm#sthash.nZW6cOOe.dpuf Accessed by April 20th, 2014.

[3] WHO. Supplement to the 2013 consolidated guidelines on the use of antiretroviral drugs for treating and preventing HIV infection. Recommendations for a public health approach.

[4] Kilby JM, Lee HY, Hazelwood JD, et al. Treatment response in acute/early infection versus advanced AIDS: equivalent fi rst and second phases of HIV RNA decline. AIDS 2008; 22: 957–62.

[5] Evans D. HIV test and treat: challenges to overcome. March 10, 2011. Available at: www.aidsmeds.com/articles/hiv_test_treat_2581_20054.shtml. Accessed April 21, 2014.

[6] Cohen MS, Chen YQ, McCauley M, et al. Prevention of HIV-1 infection with early antiretroviral therapy. New Engl J Med 2011; 365:493–505.

[7] Del Romero J. Combined antiretroviral treatment and heterosexual transmission of HIV-1: cross sectional and prospective cohort study. BMJ 2010; 340:c2205.

[8] Donnell D, Baeten JM, Kiarie J, et al. Heterosexual HIV-1 transmission after initiation of antiretroviral therapy: a prospective cohort analysis. Lancet 2010; 375:2092–8.

[9] Marks G, Crepaz N, Senterfitt JW, Janssen RS. Meta-analysis of highrisk sexual behavior in persons aware and unaware they are infected with HIV in the United States: implications for HIV prevention programs. JAIDS 2005; 39:446–53.

[10] Marks G, Crepaz N, Janssen RS. Estimating sexual transmission of HIV from persons aware and unaware that they are infected with the virus in the USA. AIDS 2006; 20:1447–50.

[11] Baggaley RF, Garnett GP, Ferguson NM. Modelling the impact of antiretroviral use in resource-poor settings. PLoS Med 2006; 3:e124.

[12]. Blower SM, Gershengorn HB, Grant RM. A tale of two futures: HIV and antiretroviral therapy in San Francisco. Science 2000; 287: 650–4.

[13] Law MG, Prestage G, Grulich A, Van de Ven P, Kippax S. Modelling the effect of combination antiretroviral treatments on HIV incidence. AIDS 2001; 15:1287–94.

[14] Brown LB, Miller WC, Kamanga G, et al. HIV partner notification is effective and feasible in sub-Saharan Africa: opportunities for HIV treatment and prevention. J Acquir Immune Defic Syndr. 2011 Apr 15;56(5):437-42.

[15] Granich RM, Gilks CF, Dye C, et al. Universal voluntary HIV testing with immediate antiretroviral therapy as a strategy for elimination of HIV transmission: a mathematical model. Lancet. 2009 Jan 3;373(9657):48-57.

[16] Severe P, Juste MA, Ambroise A, et al. Early versus standard antiretroviral therapy for HIV-infected adults in Haiti. N Engl J Med. 2010 Jul 15;363(3):257-65.

[17] Long EF, Brandeau ML, Owens DK. The cost-effectiveness and population outcomes of expanded HIV screening and antiretroviral treatment in the United States. Ann Intern Med 2010; 153:778–89.

[18] Walensky RP, Paltiel AD, Losina E, et al. Test and treat DC: forecasting the impact of a comprehensive HIV strategy in Washington DC. ClinInfect Dis 2010; 51:392–400.

[19] Sood N, Wagner Z, Jaycocks A, etc. Test-and-treat in Los Angeles: a mathematical model of the effects of test-and-treat for the population of men who have sex with men in Los Angeles County. Clin Infect Dis. 2013 Jun;56(12):1789-96. doi: 10.1093/cid/cit158. Epub 2013 Mar 13.

[20] Rochelle P. Walensky, Eric L. Ross, Nagalingeswaran Kumarasamy, ect. Cost-Effectiveness of HIV Treatment as Prevention in Serodiscordant Couples, The New England Journal of Medicine. 369:18. 2013.

[21] Jeffrey W Eaton, Nicolas A Menzies, John Stover, etc. How should HIV programs respond to evidence for the benefits of earlier treatment initiation? A combined analysis of twelve mathematical models, WHO/HIV/2013.56.

[22] Hecht R et al. Critical choices in financing the response to the global HIV/AIDS pandemic. Health Affairs 28 (6): 1591-1605, 2009.

[23] Resch, S., et al. (2011). Economic Returns to Investment in AIDS Treatment in Low and Middle Income Countries. PLoS ONE 6:e25310.

[24] Walensky, Rochelle P., et al. "Cost-effectiveness of HIV testing and treatment in the United States." Clinical Infectious Diseases 45.Supplement 4 (2007): S248-S254.

[25] Paltiel, A. David, et al. "Expanded screening for HIV in the United States—an analysis of cost-effectiveness." New England Journal of Medicine 352.6 (2005): 586-595.

[26] Lima, Viviane D., et al. "Expanded access to highly active antiretroviral therapy: a potentially powerful strategy to curb the growth of the HIV epidemic." Journal of Infectious Diseases 198.1 (2008): 59-67.

[27] Wagner, Bradley G., Brian J. Coburn, and Sally Blower. "Increasing survival time decreases the cost-effectiveness of using "test & treat" to eliminate HIV epidemics." Math Biosci Eng 10.5-6 (2013): 1673-86.

[28] Velasco-Hernandez JX, Gershengorn HB, Blower SM. Could widespread use of combination antiretroviral therapy eradicate HIV epidemics? Lancet Infect Dis 2002; 2:487–93

[29] Baggaley RF, Garnett GP, Ferguson NM. Modelling the impact of antiretroviral use in resource-poor settings. PLoS Med 2006; 3:e124.

[30] Furtures Institute. http://futureartcosts.futuresinstitute.org/artmodel.aspx?left=1&right=2. Accessed by April 20th, 2014.

[31] Sood N, Wagner Z, Jaycocks A, etc. Test-and-treat in Los Angeles: a mathematical model of the effects of test-and-treat for the population of men who have sex with men in Los Angeles County. Clin Infect Dis. 2013 Jun;56(12):1789-96.

[32] A. Gonzalez-Serna, V. D. Lima, J. S. Montaner, P. R. Harrigan, and C. J. Brumme. "Test-and-Treat" Strategy for Control of HIV and AIDS Can Lead to a Decrease, Not an Increase, of Multidrug- Resistant Viruses. CID 2013:57 (1 August).

[33] WHO HIV Drug Resistance Report, http://apps.who.int/iris/bitstream/10665/75183/1/9789241503938_eng.pdf

[34] WHO, country cooperation strategy at a glance (Botswana). 2009.

[35] National AIDS Coordinating. 2008.

[36] Krishnaswamy, S., The effects of HIV on Botswana's development progress.

[37] WHO, Global update on HIV treatment 2013: Results, Impact and Opportunities, 2013, June

[38] Gentleman R C, Lawless J F, Lindsey J C, et al. Multi-state Markov models for analysing incomplete disease history data with illustrations for hiv disease[J]. Statistics in medicine, 1994, 13(8): 805-821.

[39] Government of Botswana. The fourth Botswana HIV/AIDS Impact Survey IV (BAIS VI), 2014.

[40] Dodd, P. J., Garnett, G. P., & Hallett, T. B. (2010). Examining the promise of HIV elimination by'test and treat'in hyperendemic settings. AIDS (London, England), 24(5), 729-735.

[41] Charlebois ED, Das M, Porco TC, Havlir DV. The effect of expanded antiretroviral treatment strategies on the HIV epidemic among men who have sex with men in San Francisco. Clin Infect Dis 2011; 52: 1046–9.

[42] Sorensen, Stephen W., et al. "A mathematical model of comprehensive test-and-treat services and HIV incidence among men who have sex with men in the United States." PloS one 7.2 (2012): e29098.

[43] Lodi, Sara, et al. "Time from human immunodeficiency virus seroconversion to reaching CD4+ cell count thresholds< 200,< 350, and< 500 cells/mm3: assessment of need following changes in treatment guidelines." Clinical infectious diseases 53.8 (2011): 817-825..

[44] Helleberg, M., Kronborg, G., Larsen, C., Pedersen, G., Pedersen, C., Obel, N. and Gerstoft, J. (2013), No change in viral set point or CD4 cell decline among antiretroviral treatment-naïve, HIV-1-infected individuals enrolled in the Danish HIV Cohort Study in 1995–2010. HIV Medicine, 14: 362–369.

[45] Fasawe, Olufunke, et al. "Cost-effectiveness analysis of option B+ for HIV prevention and treatment of mothers and children in Malawi." PloS one 8.3 (2013): e57778.

[46] Raffaele Vardavas and Sally Blower. The emergence of hiv transmitted resistance in botswana: "when will the who detection threshold be exceeded?" PLoS One, 2(1):e152, 2007.

[47] Little, S. J., Holte, S., Routy, J. P.,etc. (2002). Antiretroviral-drug resistance among patients recently infected with HIV. New England Journal of Medicine, 347(6), 385-394.

[48] Farahani, M., Vable, A., Lebelonyane, R., Seipone, K., etc. (2014). Outcomes of the Botswana national HIV/AIDS treatment program from 2002 to 2010: a longitudinal analysis. The Lancet Global Health, 2(1), e44-e50.

[49] Hayes R, Sabapathy K, Fidler S. Universal testing and treatment as an HIV prevention strategy: research questions and methods [J]. Current HIV research, 2011, 9(6): 429-445.

[50] Predictors of Delayed Antiretroviral Therapy Initiation, Mortality, and Loss to Follow-up in HIV Infected Patients Eligible for HIV Treatment: Data from an HIV Cohort Study in India

[51] Government of Botswana. The Models of Care, 2012. Final Report.

[52] USAIDS. Transitional Financing and the Response to HIV/AIDS in Botswana: A country analysis. http://www.healthpolicyinitiative.com/Publications/Documents/1556_1_Botswana_Transitional_ Financing_Report.pdf. Accessed by April 25, 2014.

[53] Cleary, S. M., McIntyre, D., & Boulle, A. M. (2008). Assessing efficiency and costs of scaling up HIV treatment. AIDS, 22, S35-S42.

[54] Bruce R. Schackman, Sue J. Goldie, Kenneth A. Freedberg, ect. Comparison of Health State Utilities Using Community and Patient Preference Weights Derived from a Survey of Patients with HIV/AIDS, Med Decis Making 2002 22: 27.

[55] Gold MR, Siegel JE, Russel LB, Weinstein MC. Cost-effectiveness in health and medicine. New York, NY: Oxford University Press; 1996.

[56] Hutubessy, Raymond, Dan Chisholm, and Tessa TT Edejer. "Generalized cost-effectiveness analysis for national-level priority-setting in the health sector." Cost effectiveness and resource allocation 1.1 (2003): 8.

[57] Trading Economics. http://www.tradingeconomics.com/botswana/gdp-per-capita-ppp-us-dollar-wb-data.html. Accessed by April 16th.